The
Type 1 Life
for Adults

A Road Map for Adults with Newly Diagnosed Type 1 Diabetes

Cover by Jess Creatives
Edited by Jodi Brandon Editorial

For more information, visit www.thetype1life.com.

ISBN: 978-0-578-64926-9
Library of Congress Control Number: 2020904417

Disclaimer: The information provided within is for general informational purposes only. The author has made every effort to include information up-to-date and correct, but there are no representations or warranties, express or implied, about the completeness, accuracy, reliability, suitability, or availability with respect to the information, products, services, or related graphics contained within. Any use of this information is at your own risk.

Dedication

To my mom, dad, and sister: thank you for continuously going the extra mile for me over the last 29 years.

Table of Contents

Preface

...

When you were diagnosed, your doctors had plenty of medical information to share with you. You learned how to handle low blood sugars, count carbohydrates, and give insulin. But, maybe your doctor didn't give you information about day-to-day life with Type 1 diabetes—like how to tell your coworkers about Type 1 diabetes or how to handle traveling abroad.

I had a conversation with a doctor once about some struggles I was having, and she said, "I get it! Well, actually, *I don't.*" She knew what I was talking about because she talks to patients with Type 1 diabetes all day. But, she knows she doesn't *truly* understand the struggles, because she doesn't have Type 1 diabetes herself.

I've had Type 1 diabetes for 26 years, so it's second nature to me. My hope is that this book will provide some perspective on how to handle day-to-day life with your new diagnosis. I'm writing this guide for you, with the hope that it gives you insight and peace of mind.

In this book, you'll find many of my own experiences sprinkled in, as well as stories from other individuals with Type 1 diabetes, to give you some real-life examples. Type 1 diabetes can be messy, much like the cover of this book depicts. Every family is different, so you might not experience all of the same things and your family might handle things differently.

A Type 1 diagnosis can be scary and overwhelming for you, but in time, you'll find your groove and find that it's manageable. Having diabetes over the last 26 years has not held me back from traveling, getting married, or running my own business. Thanks to modern medicine, Type 1 diabetes is not a death sentence.

Lastly, the content in this book is not meant to be or replace medical advice. Always listen to your doctors instructions when it comes to your health.

Chapter 1
A New Normal

...

A Barbie corvette.

That's the only thing I remember about the time I spent in the hospital after being diagnosed with Type 1 diabetes. I was barely 3 years old, and it was July 4, 1993. My parents, on the other hand, remember feeling completely overwhelmed—similar to what you may be feeling.

Because I was so young, I couldn't exactly say *glucometer*. Early on, my parents named my glucometer George. I don't know if they intended for the name to stick, but up until I left for college, our entire family called it George. Naming the glucometer George made things a little less scary for me as a child and a little easier to talk about in public places. "Did you grab George?" they would ask as we headed out the door. "Have you checked George?" they would ask before we started eating dinner at a restaurant.

George was just part of my everyday life! As I'm writing this, I've had diabetes for 26 years, but it feels like I was born with diabetes. That's 26 years of insulin shots, counting calories and carbs, eating honey and glucose tabs, feeling nauseous from high blood sugars, and countless doctor appointments. No "off" switch, no remission, no breaks. And as much as I try to stay in control, there is still the very real possibility of developing complications down the road.

Getting Organized

Managing Type 1 diabetes requires a certain level of organization due to all of the different supplies, prescriptions, and doctor's appointments. You don't want to put yourself in the position of being out of insulin on a Friday night when no pharmacies are open. So, here are a few ways you can stay organized and prepared.

Utilize Auto-Refill Options

Many companies and pharmacies now have an option for customers to enroll in an auto-reorder program for their supplies. My pump and CGM supplies arrive at my door every few months, without me having to do anything. My pharmacy texts me when I have test strips or insulin ready to pick up.

Set Calendar Reminders

If you don't have the option for auto-reorder, or don't like the idea of auto-billing, set calendar reminders. If you don't already have a digital calendar you love, Google Calendar makes it easy to create a recurring event at whatever length of time works for you. Make sure to leave enough time for processing and shipping.

Give Everything its Place

It's easy to misplace your keys or wallet. But you don't want that to happen with your insulin or glucometer. I recommend giving everything its place (in your home, in your purse, at work, etc.). All of my prescriptions and supplies have their own storage space in our bedroom closet, and I leave my glucometer in the same place on our kitchen counter.

Save Necessary Contact Information

Trust me: You want to save your endocrinologist's contact information, as well as your pharmacy's and medical suppliers' contact information, in your phone. When you get an unexpected bill, or the pharmacy says you don't have any refills left, you want all this contact information handy. And if you're like me and don't like to answer calls from unknown numbers, you can avoid missing calls from your doctor or pharmacy since they'll be in your contact list.

Be Prepared

Diabetes does not care what you're doing or where you are, so you always need to be prepared—even if you're just running to the grocery store on a Tuesday night. It's easy to think about being prepared for low blood sugars at home, but you want to be prepared when driving or at work, too. I keep a bin in my car all the time with low blood sugar treatment options, and I keep a small bin at my desk as well.

Dealing with Low and High Blood Sugars

As you've probably already experienced, words can't entirely describe what low blood sugars feel like. They're scary, because you feel empty inside. You want to lie down and curl into a ball. Having low blood sugar almost feels like an out-of-body experience. You can't think clearly or make good judgments. You get easily sidetracked, confused, angry, panicky, and shaky. You may even seem drunk to those around you. Even if your blood sugar comes back up, it's not uncommon for your body to still feel low, often for another half hour.

The further you get into your diagnosis, you may experience new symptoms. You'll hear about many common symptoms from doctors, but everyone is different and can have their own symptoms. Over the years, I've heard of hypoglycemic symptoms, such as seeing white spots, ringing in the ears, sensitivity to light, feeling itchy, hallucinating, lips feeling tingly, or tongue going numb. Many people with diabetes feel confused, and I've heard extreme confusion stories from other adults like not knowing where they were, not recognizing their own house or belongings, and even momentarily thinking their spouse was having an affair.

For example, one of the patterns that my parents noticed when I was in junior high is that the weather affects my blood sugars. It sounds silly, and I've never had a doctor who believes me, but it rings true to this day as an adult. Day-to-day weather doesn't really affect me (unless it's 110 degrees outside), but the seasons changing wreaks havoc. Every year, the one- or two-week transition from fall to winter, and from spring to summer, causes my blood sugars to go haywire.

My parents also noticed a very specific symptom that signaled a low blood sugar: The circles under my eyes darken. This is not something that doctors said would happen or is even listed as a common symptom of Type 1 diabetics. My parents also noticed I would become really irritable, which signaled that I was probably low. (Maybe not every time: Sometimes I was just being a teenager.) You may have your own unusual symptoms as well.

Karen Bonar, whose father has Type 1 diabetes, remembers him going low while at Disneyland with their family. After a full day of walking and family fun, and as they were on the train headed back to the hotel, her father's blood sugar dropped. Karen recalled him not being the most compliant person while low, and he started to push Karen's mom away when she tried to give him honey. Slowly and discreetly, people near them on the train inched away. When her dad still would not take anything for his low blood sugar, and became more disgruntled, people began openly avoiding "the drunk." For Karen, it was definitely embarrassing because people thought her dad (who does not drink) had become intoxicated at Disneyland!

There are many ways to treat your low blood sugar. Growing up, having a Capri Sun juice was my go-to remedy at home. I secretly enjoyed going low when we were out getting groceries or watching my sister's volleyball games because it usually meant I could get a regular can of soda to bring up my blood sugar. I've also treated my lows with glucose tabs, cake frosting, honey, Jolly Ranchers, and Smarties. (Once, I had a doctor who had me try slow, deep breathing during a low blood sugar to bring my levels up. It didn't work.)

While a can of regular soda was a rare "treat" for going low, the best (and worst) was going low in the middle of the night. If you haven't heard about it yet, there is a bit of an inside joke within the diabetes community about how much we eat during middle-of-the-night lows. Growing up, I always went for tortillas. I don't know why we always seemed to have them, but we did! In college, I didn't have much "extra" food around my apartment to snack on during a 2 a.m. low, so I ended up eating broccoli. (It didn't help.)

Then, there are high blood sugars. High blood sugars aren't usually such an extreme experience in terms of symptoms. Typically they cause nausea and thirst, but there is the risk of your high blood sugar leading to developing ketones or diabetic ketoacidosis (DKA)—which might even be how you found out you had Type 1 diabetes in the first place. Ketones occur when the body doesn't have enough insulin. Left untreated, it can lead to DKA. I have been lucky enough to not experience this myself, but in simple terms, DKA happens when your body lacks insulin and begins producing extra blood acids. Your doctor should talk with you in-depth about how this happens, what to look for, and what to do if you develop DKA.

As a result of long-term high blood sugars, you may also experience a false sense of hypoglycemia. I've experienced this when my blood sugars were predominantly in the upper 100s and 200s for several months. As you work to regulate your blood sugars, you may deal with this false sense of hypoglycemia. Your body may make you feel like you are experiencing a low blood sugar when, really, your blood sugar is only 150. It's a very frustrating experience: You can't drink juice to remedy a false low blood sugar, because you are not actually low. Eventually, your body will adjust to the new normal (where it should be), and the feeling will subside.

Occasionally, you may also get on the blood sugar roller coaster—and it's not fun. The roller coaster begins when you take too much insulin for a big meal, and then your blood sugar goes low. You happen to over-treat your low blood sugar with too much juice or candy, and as a result, an hour later, your blood sugar goes high. So, you take too much insulin, and once again, your blood sugar goes low. And the cycle continues. Hopefully, you don't over-treat a second time, or take too much insulin again, but it can happen.

At the end of the day, remember that diabetes does not own you. Nor does it define you. This is hard to remember, because Type 1 diabetes is a 24-hours-a-day, all-consuming condition.

Recognizing Patterns

A new diagnosis is stressful because everything feels overwhelming. There is so much new information to remember and so many numbers to track. The bad news is that diabetes can be unpredictable. You might do the same thing two days in a row and get different results. The good news is, despite the unpredictability, you will hopefully and eventually start to notice patterns.

Immediately after a diagnosis, you might also be in what's called a "honeymoon period" with your diabetes. No honeymoon period is exactly the same, but in essence, it can almost seem like your blood sugars are great without any insulin at all. You'll want to stay in close contact with your doctor during this time—and this could last anywhere from a few weeks to several months.

Your doctor likely discussed this with you, but if not, it's important to keep track of your blood sugars in a physical logbook, or on an app, and make notes with each blood sugar check or insulin dosage. At the end of each week or month, review this data. You might see that your weekly family pizza night is raising your blood sugar, or that your blood sugar runs higher on stressful days at work. This is something you should continue to do long-term, because patterns may change and new patterns may develop.

To help identify patterns, set a consistent schedule. This schedule may not be possible all of the time with work activities and traveling, but adhering to a some type of schedule reduces the number of variables in what feels like a never-ending science experiment called Type 1 diabetes. Without a consistent schedule, it'll be harder to determine which specific foods or activities are causing any high or low blood sugars.

Thanks to modern technology, there are three types of smartphone apps that can benefit individuals with Type 1 diabetes: blood sugar logs, carbohydrate counters, and continuous glucose monitoring apps. Each category has variations, and more apps are being developed every year, but I want to highlight some of the more popular types of apps to get you started.

Blood Sugar Logs
Growing up, I had to write down my blood sugars on paper, but today we can keep track of everything digitally. MySugr: Diabetes Tracker Log and Glucose Buddy Diabetes Tracker allow you to track blood sugar levels, record insulin intake, track carbs, and track any other miscellaneous info you want to track with regard to your health. Though both apps have free versions, you can pay a small fee per month for additional features.

Some glucometers also have a smartphone app: Accu-Chek® Aviva Connect, CONTOUR® NEXT ONE, Dario Smart Glucose Meter, One Drop | Chrome, and OneTouch Verio Flex®, to name a few. Each of the meters connects with the app, making it easy to review blood sugars and share data. These glucometers and apps save you the trouble of having to remember to manually log your blood sugars.

Carbohydrate Counters

Whether you're eating out or at a friend's house, you will often be in situations in which you don't know the exact calorie or carbohydrate count of a particular food. Plenty of apps allow you to search nutrition facts for foods, but MyFitnessPal and CalorieKing are two that I recommend. Both apps also have the option to upgrade for additional features.

Continuous Glucose Monitoring Apps

If you have a continuous glucose monitor (also known as a CGM, which I'll talk about later in this book), there are a few apps that you can download to use in conjunction with the CGM. To start, Dexcom has an iPhone app to act as the CGM receiver. You can also download apps like Sugarmate to enable more notifications or Diabits to get blood sugar predictions based on your activity. Neither of these apps has the option to upgrade.

Different Factors that Affect Blood Sugars

High blood sugars, low blood sugars, and everything in between—what can cause your blood sugars to fluctuate? Obviously, food and insulin are the biggest factors. But many other things can impact blood sugar levels. Some of these may not ever affect you, or may do so only temporarily, but they are things to be aware of, just in case. Keep in mind this is not an exhaustive list, and you can talk to a registered dietitian or diabetes specialist about your specific situation.

Specific Foods
You may find that anytime you eat a particular food or meal, your blood sugar skyrockets. High-carb foods like pizza and pasta seem to affect a lot of people with Type 1 diabetes, but there's a chance those foods won't affect you. Other foods that have been known to cause issues for some individuals include oatmeal, applesauce, and even drinks with caffeine. It's totally a case-by-case basis, so you'll just need to watch for patterns.

You'll notice that some people with Type 1 diabetes will eat whatever they want, and take insulin to "cover" it, while other individuals avoid foods with sugars. To figure out what types of foods you can or cannot eat on a day-to-day basis, talk with your doctor. Your "diet" may be more strict at the beginning of your diagnosis as you and your doctor figure out your insulin ratios.

Holidays

During special occasions like holidays or family reunions, people tend to eat more. It's also pretty likely that your family doesn't eat your "typical" (everyday) foods for holidays and other special occasions. With different foods and bigger portions, the holidays can cause some problems with your blood sugars. Talk to your doctor about how to prepare for the holidays and what you should or should not eat. Your doctor may have you increase your long-acting insulin or increase your basal rates on your insulin pump.

Emotions

The first week at a new job can be exciting and stressful for any one, and individuals with Type 1 diabetes can have a harder time during this first week. Any stressful, emotional, or high-pressure situation can cause some blood sugar issues. Whether it's a breakup, preparing for a big presentation at work, losing a pet, fighting with friends or family, or changing jobs, be prepared for fluctuating blood sugars.

Being Sick

Whether it's a head cold or the flu, being sick is another factor that can affect your blood sugars. It's extra stress on the body, not to mention that you are probably not eating as much and might be dehydrated. Some medicines (both over-the-counter and prescription) can also raise your blood sugars. Be sure to talk with your doctor before taking any medicine and discuss how to handle your sickness.

Alcohol

According to the American Diabetes Association, alcohol can cause a drop in blood sugar levels. Because of the impact that alcohol has on blood sugars, it's important for you to eat something along with alcohol and check your blood sugar more often than usual after drinking. It can get a little more complicated if your drink has lots of sugar in it, like a margarita or daiquiri, as the alcohol lowers blood sugar levels but the sugar raises levels. It's taken some trial and error for me to figure out the best solution for me; consult your doctor for specific advice.

Doctors recommend that you wear some type of diabetes identification in general, but especially when you may be drinking alcohol. The symptoms of too much alcohol and a low blood sugar can be similar, and you don't want friends (or strangers) brushing you off as just being too intoxicated. For this reason, I've always made sure that I'm not alone during or after drinking. (You can find medical identification resources at www.thetype1life.com.)

Action Steps

1. Set aside an afternoon this week to get organized. Call to set up auto-refills, add calendar reminders, put supplies in your car, etc.

2. Decide how you will track your blood sugars and how often you will sit down to review the data. If you use a digital calendar, like Google Calendar, it's easy to make a recurring event reminder each month to review your data.

3. Download and test out any of the apps mentioned in this chapter, and decide if you want to add them into your routine.

Chapter 2
Doctors, Medical Supplies, and Insurance

...

The door was closed, but I remember hearing his voice bellow loudly as he talked to the patient. It was obvious that the patient in the room was not managing their diabetes like they should.

After hearing this, I didn't want to go in—much less by myself.

My mom was with me, but since I was in middle school, she wanted me to start going into the exam room alone—to be more independent. Dr. Guthrie was my endocrinologist from the very start, and even with his big hugs, I always felt timid around him. He was a doctor who meant business, and he knew when his patients weren't doing what we were supposed to do.

Dr. Guthrie was so good that we sometimes drove two hours just to see him for a half-hour appointment. As a child, I didn't fully understand how great a doctor he was, or even the importance of a great doctor. It didn't hit me until college, when I had to switch doctors. For about six years, I struggled to find a decent endocrinologist. I ran into some doctors who weren't a great fit for me, for varying reasons:

- One told me I was healthy and beautiful when I asked about how to lose weight as someone with Type 1 diabetes.
- One seemed to have an anger problem.
- One didn't even look at my blood sugars, instead asked me how I was feeling, and wanted to adjust my insulin settings based on that alone.
- Another also didn't look at my blood sugars and spent the least amount of time with me of any other doctor I've visited.

If there's one thing my mom taught me, and something that I hope you also remember, it's that *you have to be your own best advocate.* We drove two hours because Dr. Guthrie was the best, and he was worth it. It's okay to challenge your doctor, or to go to two different doctors in a year.

One of the hardest parts of being an individual with diabetes is never feeling like you're doing enough. It feels like so many variables are out of your control, so doctor appointments are not always enjoyable because you are scrutinized and given a list of things to work on.

When my friend Ellie Hook, who has had Type 1 diabetes for more than 20 years, was in college, she went to an endocrinologist appointment in which her new doctor said, "Wow, you're working really hard to manage your disease. I see you check consistently, but your blood sugars are all over the board. As you know, that's totally normal for adolescents. We can make a modification here since you're trending high at this time." As a diabetic, it is very rare to actually have a doctor acknowledge our hard work and not blame. All individuals deserve this type of care from their doctors, but it's not always a reality.

What to Look For

You will be seeing your endocrinologist and diabetes care team regularly, so you want people you can fully trust with your health.

While I do reference endocrinologists in this book, many patients with Type 1 diabetes are instead seen by a nurse practitioner and a diabetes educator. In some offices, the endocrinologist is the primary provider of information, and you only see a diabetes educator or dietician on occasion. Other times, most of the diabetes care is carried out by a diabetes nurse specialist or nurse practitioner, under the care of an endocrinologist. Either route is fine, as long as you are happy with the standard of care.

The hospital may have referred you to someone, and it's fine to stick with that doctor. In fact, you may love him or her! The following factors are things to keep in mind in the future, should you ever need a new doctor.

Availability
When you call to make an appointment, how booked is the doctor? Having to wait six months is not a good sign. You want to find some middle ground (say, one to three months). If you can't see someone for six months, it likely means they are overbooked. When a doctor is overbooked, your appointment may start late, and you may feel rushed during the appointment. There are several things to cover in an appointment, so you want adequate time to discuss everything with your doctor. Also, ask the doctor if you can call with questions or submit blood sugars between appointments. Most doctors want to see their patients every three to four months.

Changes

Thanks to research, we have so much information about how to handle diabetes through a variety of scenarios. With the help of technology, managing diabetes has become incredibly easier. But, even with research and technology, there are still hiccups in controlling blood sugars and being a healthy individual. Is your doctor open to trying new things, like new medicines or devices? I kept asking doctors for advice on losing weight, to no avail. Finally, when I asked a new doctor this same question, I was given a few options. My doctor didn't push these options on me, and she laid out the pros and cons of each.

Questions and Discussion

Your doctor should allow you to ask questions and address any issues. (If you ever feel an issue is urgent, call the doctor's office; do not wait until the next appointment.) In my experience, doctors who are overbooked and rushed usually want to do the bare minimum. As I've mentioned, many factors affect blood sugars, so you need to discuss these with your doctor. Some things you might want to discuss at each appointment are:

- New symptoms or problems you've noticed (even if unrelated to diabetes).
- Any major changes that have occurred since your last visit.
- New medications that you have started taking.
- Updates to family medical history.

Data

Since I mentioned it previously, you probably expected this to make the list: Doctors need to actually look at blood sugars. I used to have to write down all of my blood sugars in a log book and bring it to appointments, but now it's as easy as letting the doctor download your blood sugars from your glucometer. Once they've downloaded your glucometer, they can look at averages, patterns, before-meal levels, after-meal levels, and more. From there, they will make any necessary adjustments to insulin levels and ratios. (Some offices prefer that you download or send this data ahead of time, so be sure to ask for the doctor's preference if they don't mention it.)

Overall Health

Appointments usually start with checking your height, weight, and blood pressure. The doctor should be asking about your overall health and communicating any updates with your other doctors. If there are any concerning reports or notes from other doctors, they will discuss them at your appointment. Also, endocrinologists generally check your feet to make sure there aren't signs of neuropathy.

Blood Work

A few times each year, you will need to have blood drawn and provide a urine sample. The best scenario is having the tests done a week before your appointment with the doctor (so they can review the results with you). Often, though, you will have blood work done after an appointment, and they will just call you with results. The doctor will look at a variety of things, but the one result talked about the most is the A1C. The A1C test shows the average blood sugar levels over the past three months. Based on those results, your doctor will make adjustments to your insulin and food ratios, if needed. (I always describe this to people without Type 1 diabetes as my diabetes grade point average, or GPA.)

Other Doctors

You'll most often visit an endocrinologist, the doctor who assists in the actual management of your diabetes. As an individual with diabetes, optimal health requires a team of doctors. You will need to visit these doctors regularly, if you aren't already.

Eye Doctor
People with diabetes who struggle with high blood sugars are at risk for damaged blood vessels in the retina, commonly referred to as diabetic retinopathy. It cannot be cured, only prevented with good blood sugar management. You want to be sure your blood sugars are in good control during the day of each eye exam so that results are accurate.

Dentist

People with diabetes are also at a higher risk for gum disease when blood sugars are not controlled. Regular visits to the dentist are important to keep teeth clean and to stay on top of any infections that may develop.

Podiatrist

Another common complication associated with Type 1 diabetes is neuropathy, because people with diabetes are prone to poor blood flow and nerve damage. It's unlikely you will need to see a podiatrist regularly, unless the endocrinologist notices a problem and refers you to one.

Insulin Pumps and Continuous Glucose Monitors

Your doctor may recommend that you try using an insulin pump. I remember seeing an insulin pump for the first time at a summer camp for children with Type 1 diabetes. I was still in grade school at the time, so the doctors and education staff weren't getting too technical with us yet. I remember thinking that the few campers who did have an insulin pump had something "extra wrong" with them. (Clearly, I hadn't been fully educated on what an insulin pump is and why it is so beneficial to people with Type 1 diabetes.)

I didn't get my first insulin pump until I was a senior in high school, once the price had come down, and we had good insurance coverage. Not a single classmate teased me about my insulin pump. In fact, many of them thought it was really interesting. The only exception was the junior high student who thought my insulin pump was an mp3 player, and asked why I got to bring my mp3 player to school and he didn't.

An insulin pump can easily fit into pant pockets, so it's typically not too visible. Most of the time, if someone notices it, it's because they are either diabetic themselves or have someone close to them who has an insulin pump.

Having an insulin pump is not cheap, but the convenience is so worth it, in my opinion. I've now had my insulin pump for more than 10 years, and it's hard to imagine going back to multiple daily injections. The pump has two main functions: boluses and basal rates. A bolus is taken with food, or to correct high blood sugars. A basal rate is background insulin, similar to how an IV slowly administers medicine, to keep blood sugar levels more consistent throughout the day. Some patients eventually choose to take a break from their insulin pump, though, because they don't want to stay tethered to a device forever.

Here are a few considerations when deciding whether to get an insulin pump:

- Wearing an insulin pump means you won't have to carry around a needle and bottle of insulin. When eating at a restaurant, you wouldn't have to try to be discreet or go to the restroom to take your insulin.
- Insulin pumps can deliver more accurate and specific insulin dosages. For example, with insulin injections, you can take 12 units; with an insulin pump, 12.7 units. Individuals can also use square or dual-wave boluses, which spread out the bolus over a specified amount of time.
- Individuals can obtain greater control of their blood sugars with varied basal rates. For example, for optimal blood sugar levels, my doctor and I have set six different basal rates throughout the day. One of the morning basal rates is lower, because I work out in the mornings, and it lessens the chance of my blood sugar going low.

While we're talking about insulin pumps, it's also important to briefly talk about continuous glucose monitors (CGMs), because they are often purchased and used together (though they don't have to be). Your doctor will likely discuss this with you, but if they haven't yet, a CGM is a small sensor inserted into the skin that continuously provides insight into glucose levels.

What's really great about having a CGM is that it sends updates to a receiver or your smartphone every few minutes, so you constantly know what your blood sugar levels are. It will sound a small alarm if your blood sugars are rapidly rising or falling, so you can be aware that you may need treatment soon. I use a Dexcom sensor, and I have the ability to send certain alerts to my husband's phone. Since I run my own business and work alone from my home, this extra alert feature provides some peace of mind for my husband and me.

Doctors are typically advocates of CGMs because you can really keep tighter control of blood sugars. I didn't get a CGM until a few years after college, when my doctor recommended it to improve my blood sugar control. It can also turn into a roundabout way for individuals to gamify Type 1 diabetes care. People post pictures of their daily graph on social media, bragging about how they were finally able to stay within a certain range for a certain amount of time.

Troubleshooting

As great as they are, insulin pumps don't come without their problems! I've definitely had my fair share of annoyances and had to figure out what to do with my insulin pump in different scenarios. Even though pumps come with a manual, and you will undergo training with your doctor before you start wearing it, here's some insight on troubleshooting common problems that come with an insulin pump.

One of the first things to note is that you need to rotate your pump site. The pump reservoir and site need to be changed every two to three days. You want to be sure to rotate the location of your site. Just like with insulin shots, tissue can build up under the skin if a site is in the same spot too often. I try to do a rotation: left side of the stomach, right side of the stomach, left leg, right leg, and so on. If you don't rotate enough, it can affect insulin absorption.

As can any technology, pumps can sometimes quit at the most inopportune times. (For me, one of those times was during my husband's and my move into our first house!) There's no warning; the pump simply starts buzzing or beeping, and displays an error message. Sometimes it's an error message to do with the reservoir, and other times the screen freezes and the pump stops completely.

If your insulin pump goes on the fritz, and you need to get a new one, there are two things to do. First, call your insulin pump company and report the issue. They'll ask you a few questions to confirm that it does need to be replaced. Because these devices administer life-saving medicine, the company will prioritize replacement shipping and can usually get a new insulin pump to you within a day or two. Depending on your insurance coverage and the warranty on the pump, you may need to pay for part of the replacement. After that step, call your doctor.

Usually, the doctor will call in a prescription for a long-acting insulin for you to take until your insulin pump arrives. You'll still take short-acting insulin when you eat or need to correct a high blood sugar, and then also take long-acting insulin to act as your basal rate. You'll need to go to the pharmacy to get this long-acting insulin, as well as some needles if you don't have any on hand. It's easy to keep some spare needles around, but because insulin has a relatively short shelf life, it doesn't financially make sense to keep long-acting insulin on hand at all times. (You can also buy NPH insulin at the pharmacy without a prescription.)

Again, these insulin pump malfunctions aren't too common and, though annoying, can be easily handled.

The Emotional Toll of Insulin Pumps

My sister didn't like the idea of me getting an insulin pump in high school. It made my invisible disease more visible. Insulin pumps can come with their occasional technical problems, as well as an emotional and mental toll. Even after being on an insulin pump for more than 10 years, though, the downsides are outweighed by the benefit of being on an insulin pump.

Getting an insulin pump also requires an internal adjustment period. Though it's not painful, it is a new experience to be attached or tethered to a device at all times. Through trial and error, you'll figure out how to wear your pump when sleeping, while playing sports, and when wearing clothes without pockets, and what to do at special occasions like a wedding. It should only take a few times for the tubing to catch on a doorknob and pull out the pump site for you to learn to hide the excess tubing in your pocket! Because insulin pumps are so popular now, there are actually plenty of insulin pump accessories: covers, pouches, cases, and more.

At the end of the day, there's no right or wrong way to feel about your insulin pump. Over time, all the data intake and the site changes may be too much, and you may want to take a break from it.

Dealing with Insurance and Supply Companies

In addition to doctors, you'll also be interacting a lot with insurance companies and medical supply companies—especially if you have an insulin pump or continuous glucose monitor (CGM).

I can't tell you the number of times that my insurance company has sent me a letter announcing that it will no longer cover something that I use. I've had to change insulin brands, needles, and glucometers many times over the years. For me, and many others, the most frustrating part is that insurance often changes again, causing you to switch back, sometimes less than a year later.

Having to deal with insurance so often is part of why it's so important to have a great doctor. You want a doctor, or a doctor's staff, who is responsive and willing to submit paperwork (sometimes repeatedly) to your insurance provider so you can get the supplies you need.

Here are a few quick tips for calling insurance or medical supply companies:

- Try to call first thing in the morning when representatives haven't been hounded all day.
- Take notes during your call.
- Get the name and number of the person with whom you spoke.
- If possible, get confirmation numbers for orders or claims submitted.

If (or when) your insurance won't cover a particular brand of insulin or device, petition them for an exception. You and your doctor will need to send in a letter of medical necessity, explaining why you believe the company should cover your particular needs. This process can take weeks or even months.

Based on what insurance and medical companies have had me write before, your letter of medical necessity should include:

- A description of your condition.
- Any challenges you have experienced with different brands.
- Your personal medical history, especially any dangerous incidents.
- Rationale for why this device or brand is needed.
- Why you would benefit from this particular device or brand.

You should also ask your doctor and insurance provider if there is anything else that needs to be included in the letter of necessity.

Switching Insurance Companies
Inevitably, you will likely switch insurance companies at least a few times in your life. There are a few details to spe-

cifically ask about when it comes to switching companies or plans:

- The deductible and out-of-pocket costs.
- Coverage for durable medical equipment (your pump and sensor).
- If durable medical equipment has a different coinsurance than other things.
- How/where pump supplies, prescriptions, test strips, and CGM supplies fit in their plan.
- Their drug/prescription formulary, as that will affect your cost on insulin.

Diabetic Alert Dogs

In addition to CGMs, many people with diabetes are beginning to utilize diabetic alert dogs. Lauren Burke was diagnosed with Type 1 diabetes when she was 12 years old. A few years later, her endocrinologist told her about diabetic alert dogs, but most organizations wouldn't place an alert dog with someone younger than 18. It wasn't until Lauren got to college that she started researching and jumping through all the hoops to try to get her own diabetic alert dog.

After Lauren graduated from college, she was placed with her current alert dog, Ricki. Ricki alerts Lauren to high blood sugars, low blood sugars, and blood sugar changes greater than 10%. Lauren finds that Ricki beats her Dexcom G6 sensor by 20+ minutes every time. Ricki alerts in real time: She smells the chemical changes in Lauren's body as they are happening, whereas CGMs wait for the blood from your core to get into your interstitial fluid.

Lauren still wears her CGM religiously, because there is so much an alert dog doesn't tell you, nor are they perfect animals. For example, an alert dog can't catch your blood sugars drifting up at 2 a.m. if it's not taking you out of your normal blood sugar range. And, Lauren has learned not to expect night alerts if she and Ricki had an overly active day.

While it might sound like a good idea to have an alert dog around, Lauren says that having an alert dog is a lot of work. Your whole lifestyle has to change to adjust and accommodate a dog. There are some things to think about, like:

- Is it really a commitment you want to make?
- Where will your dog be while the two of you are at work?
- Do you have room under your desk for a bed and a 60-pound dog?
- Are you on your feet all day?
- Will your dog have enough downtime with your busy schedule?
- Can you handle people stopping you everywhere

you go every day (in line at the grocery store, while waiting to cross a street, at work) to ask you about your dog?

It seems like an incredible thing (you can take your dog anywhere!), but you have to remember you're not taking your dog *anywhere*—you're taking your dog *everywhere*. Everywhere you go, people may point and stare at you. You'll have to tell people every day to not distract your dog, because they're working. You have to patiently educate people. Very few people assume a dog is an alert dog, and if they do, they often assume you're blind. Every day, people assume Lauren is training her dog, when in reality they've been together for more than three years.

According to Lauren, an alert dog won't make your job as a person with Type 1 diabetes much easier. A well-trained dog will be taught to never give up, and if their human doesn't act to correct an out-of-range blood sugar, the dog should go to alert more people. You can't cheat or turn the alarms off on a dog! Lauren says having a dog constantly alert you for several hours can be a lot to mentally and emotionally handle. There have been times when Lauren has gotten frustrated with her own dog, because she's already corrected her high blood sugar, but her blood sugar is not budging—and Ricki continues to alert. But you can't get mad at the dog, because they're doing their job, and this is what you want and need them to do.

If you are interested in potentially getting a diabetic alert dog, Assistance Dogs International (ADI) is the global accrediting body of service animals. ADI holds nonprofits to high standards in an effort to make sure they take good care of the consumers. ADI also partners with governments across the globe to standardize service animals and their public access rights. If your alert dog is not from an ADI-accredited organization, it can make traveling out of the country more difficult. (Each country has different laws and public access standards, so make sure to do your research before you plan your trip!)

Good organizations put in a lot of time and effort to place people with the right dog. For example, Early Alert Canines spends a whole day with each client working with each dog to make sure an appropriate match is made. Finding the right match is important, and each dog should match their human partner's energy level and lifestyle. A lazy, low-key dog wouldn't be a good match for an active, on-the-go tri-athlete, for example, and an energetic, playful dog wouldn't be a good match for a household with very young children or caring for an elderly relative.

Action Steps

1. If you have other doctors you see regularly, call those doctors' offices and let them know about your diagnosis. It may be they just make a note in your file, or they may want you to come in for an appointment.

2. If it's not in the same place where you track your blood sugars, decide where you will write down any non-urgent questions to ask at your next appointment. You might consider having one notebook in which you write down questions for your doctor, notes from calls with your insurance provider, etc.

3. Talk to your doctor about the potential of getting an insulin pump or continuous glucose monitor (CGM). Ask about the different options available for each.

4. Call your insurance provider to see if an insulin pump or continuous glucose monitor would be covered under your plan. You may want to ask if coverage would be different for different brands.

Chapter 3
Family and Support Systems

...

After your diagnosis, you'll need to tell people about your diabetes. With social media, it's easy to tell several people at once, so you can opt to do this to save time and address multiple questions at once. There are some people you'll want to have more in-depth conversations with, though, especially those who will be around you more often—neighbors, coworkers, roommates, friends, and extended family, for example.

Maybe it's not the first thing you bring up in a conversation, but there's no need to be embarrassed or ashamed of having Type 1 diabetes. It's important that you tell those around you, so that they are informed if something happens. For example, low blood sugar symptoms can sometimes be mistaken for being drunk. If you're acting funny or not making sense, your boss needs to know that you're not drunk but that you might be having a low blood sugar. Some of my closest friends even know the basics about treating low and high blood sugars.

When I had to start taking shots before lunch in grade school, my parents and I decided it was best to only tell a few of my closest friends. I had attended this school for two and a half years, so everyone knew I had Type 1 diabetes. This new information wasn't something that everyone needed to know, though, because it didn't affect them. Likewise, you don't have to tell everyone in the office about your diagnosis. You can tell more and more people as you feel comfortable.

When I went to college, I didn't tell every single person that I had Type 1 diabetes. I told the resident assistant in my dorm, my roommate, and a few of my professors. Just like in grade school, more and more people found out over time. I told them when it was appropriate or if I felt they needed to know. Many people actually found out when they saw my insulin pump, which made it easy for me to have a conversation about my diabetes.

These conversations will also involve describing the distinction between Type 1 and Type 2 diabetes. It's not uncommon for people to reference diabetes and not make the distinction between Type 1 and Type 2. Type 1 diabetes is an autoimmune disease, whereas Type 2 diabetes is usually caused by lifestyle factors or genetics. A common misconception is that if an adult is diagnosed with diabetes, it's automatically Type 2 diabetes. People with Type 1 diabetes have a pancreas that no longer produces any insulin, so they will always need to take insulin to stay alive (or at least until there is a cure). People with Type 2 diabetes have a pancreas that may produce some insulin, but not enough. People with Type 2 diabetes can usually control their diabetes with exercise, diet, and oral medications (but may need to eventually also start taking insulin). I still have to describe the difference to people and explain that I didn't get diabetes from eating too much candy.

You may have people offer you random "cures" for your Type 1 diabetes. Among the more interesting "cure myths" I've heard: exercising more, doing a cleanse, taking cinnamon pills, drinking okra or cucumber water, and using essential oils. These unusual ideas come from people who are misinformed about the differences between Type 1 and Type 2 diabetes, and how the body works.

For people who might be around you more often—like roommates or family—you may want to do some sort of informal training for them. When I was young, my mom created a booklet of diabetes information to give to teachers and babysitters. It folded horizontally, and each section had a tab with a title like low blood sugars, snacks, and glucagon treatment. It was small enough to hang on the refrigerator, and easy enough to flip to the right section when they needed to remember how much insulin to give me. You can download a template at www.thetype1life.com.

Extended Family

Growing up, holidays were pretty normal for me. I was lucky enough to have a very loving and caring extended family. On my mother's side, both of my grandparents had diabetes. Because my mom's family was accustomed to having people with diabetes in the family, it wasn't as big of a deal to have another person with Type 1 diabetes.

My mom had eight brothers and sisters, and almost everyone would gather at my grandmother's house for the holidays each year. Everyone would bring meals, desserts, and drinks to share, and several family members made sure to bring a case of Diet Coke or bake sugar-free cookies.

My dad's parents were just as great. My dad only had one brother, so we were a much smaller family. I was the only person with Type 1 diabetes on this side of the family (until recently), but that didn't matter; my grandma made sure to bake a sugar-free pie and have sugar-free ice cream on hand. My parents and grandparents would also eat the sugar-free desserts.

As a reminder, talk to your doctor about how to best handle holiday foods. Other than desserts or diet soda, not many menu additions or adjustments need to be made, unless you know a particular food wreaks havoc on your blood sugars. If you have family who is not as understanding, explain to them that, for the most part, you can still eat like other adults: lean meats, whole grains, and fruits and vegetables. Your family may not realize that you might feel excluded without sugar-free treats or drinks that you can have, so you can either have further conversations with them or bring your own treats. Or, your doctor may say that you can eat a certain amount of "regular" dessert!

(Note that many recipes can be made sugar-free by replacing sugar with Splenda or Stevia, or any other sugar substitute. Be cautious, though, about how many sugar-free sweets you consume in one sitting. If eaten too much, sugar-free treats can sometimes cause some digestive issues, and you may be spending your holiday in the bathroom.)

Online and In-Person Communities

Like many chronic illnesses, diabetes is an invisible monster. As much as we can try to describe how it feels to have a low or high blood sugar, it's something that has to be experienced to be fully understood. Because of this, finding a community of others who have Type 1 diabetes can be incredibly helpful.

One of the best experiences of my life was finding this community through attending a summer camp called Camp Discovery, a week-long camp only for children with Type 1 diabetes children and teenagers. I attended as a camper for more than 15 years and then became a camp counselor. A lot of kids come to Camp Discovery from small rural communities where they're the only one with Type 1 diabetes, so part of camp is being able to shake off that "freak" status.

Though a handful of summer camps for adults with Type 1 diabetes exist, most adults with diabetes find community with others online or in their own local community.

Facebook Groups

There is a Facebook group for just about everything. I've found groups for women with diabetes, people in my area who have diabetes, and people who use a Dexcom sensor like I do. These groups are a great place to vent frustrations or get advice from others who have experienced the same things.

Local JDRF Chapters

The Juvenile Diabetes Research Foundation (JDRF) hosts events to help raise funds to support research, education, and advocacy for individuals with Type 1 diabetes. There are a variety of events from walks and runs, bicycle races, golf competitions, and galas. Some chapters also have meetups or support groups. You can find events in your area by looking on the JDRF website. Their events are for people of all ages, not just children.

Beyond Type 1

Beyond Type 1 is a nonprofit organization that uses platforms, programs, resources, and grants to raise awareness and education about Type 1 diabetes. They have great programs to connect those with Type 1 diabetes, like a pen pal program, running teams, and biking teams.

Action Steps

1. Talk to your extended family about your diagnosis. Depending on your family situation, this could be done via email, via phone call, or in person. You may need to remind them again closer to holidays or family gatherings.
2. Join a few Facebook groups for people with Type 1 diabetes to make some friends.
3. Try to get involved in a local JDRF chapter, even if you can only attend one event a year.

Chapter 4
Dating, Marriage, and Parenting

...

I woke up and wondered why I couldn't move.

After a few minutes, I somehow forced my arm to nudge my husband, Aaron, enough to wake him. "I can't move," I told him. He was half-asleep and didn't understand what I meant, so I repeated myself and also noted that I thought my blood sugar was low.

He hurried to the kitchen to get honey and then tried to hand it to me when he walked back in. With tears streaming down my face, I told him he needed to put the honey in my mouth. I had lived 21 years with Type 1 diabetes, but I had never experienced this feeling before.

We waited for the honey to kick in and to see if I would start to feel normal again. Instead, it got worse. I tried to talk, but my speech was intermittent and slurred. I knew what I wanted to say, but the words wouldn't form. Terrified, I stared at Aaron with tears in my eyes, trying to will my mouth to move. He was equally terrified, as his wild-eyed wife just silently, and intently, stared at him, at 2 o'clock in the morning of her 25th birthday. He was truly scared, as I had never had a low blood sugar make me act that way.

Eventually, I communicated to Aaron to call my sister. I'm not sure why I wanted him to do this, as I still couldn't form words much. She urged Aaron to not wait it out, but instead to take me to the emergency room.

By the time we arrived at the ER, I was a bit more coherent. But then, things got worse again. I was acting so erratic that the doctors asked Aaron if I had taken drugs, and ordered blood work to verify that I had not. I was admitted and spent a few days in the hospital, and lots of tests were run. While the main reason I ended up there was a low blood sugar, *how* everything happened concerned the doctors.

The doctors never reached a conclusion, but they did think part of what contributed to this scary event was stress. Five months prior, I unexpectedly lost my mom in a car wreck, so I was dealing with a lot of grief and depression. This was my first birthday without my mom, and in a few weeks, I was to bury my mom's ashes. Stress has always had an effect on my blood sugars, and the doctors believed it just built up to be too much for my system.

After being discharged, I visited more doctors, in part because for several weeks after I was discharged, I couldn't eat anything and kept getting sick. I saw both a neurologist and gastroenterologist, with still no solution. For a few weeks, they thought I had gastroesophageal reflux disease (GERD), but that turned out to not be the case. To this day, we don't know for sure what happened or how I got better.

Looking back, going to these different doctors was the perfect example of me being my own advocate. If it weren't for my parents teaching me to advocate for my own health, I may not have gone through all of that to try to find answers. This experience also showed me how important it was that Aaron knew what to do.

Protecting Yourself while Living Alone

If you don't have roommates, you'll want to think about what kind of safety precautions you can take to protect yourself. I know several people with diabetes who live alone and worry about the possibility of their blood sugar dropping too low with no one there to help. Here are a few things you could do:

- Introduce yourself to your neighbors, and give one

of them a spare key into your house or apartment. You could also give a key to close friends or someone you're dating.

- Get a CGM, and have friends and family in the area "follow" your CGM through the app.
- If you don't have a CGM, implement your own routine in which you text your blood sugar to a family member or friend every morning and evening. (If they don't hear from you, that could indicate to them that something might be wrong.)
- Wear a Life Alert® necklace around the house.
- Make sure to have low blood sugar treatment supplies in various places around your house or apartment, so you're never too far away from them.

Dating and Marriage

Diabetes is a life-altering disease. You can live a happy, fulfilling life with it, no doubt. But it *is* something that requires a lot of attention to detail. When I was younger, I remember wondering if there would be a man who would even want to have a wife with Type 1 diabetes.

Some people are very open and up-front about their diabetes, to the point of listing it in their online dating profile. Other people don't tell until after a few dates. It's really up to you!

I don't remember the specific details of how I told my husband, Aaron, that I have Type 1 diabetes. I do remember having some conversations with him early on, during which he asked lots of questions about my diabetes. It never seemed to phase him in the slightest. From Aaron's perspective, marrying someone with diabetes was never intimidating or scary. We dated for two years, so we had plenty of conversations about the ups and downs of diabetes. Because I was honest and transparent about my diabetes, his expectations and the reality of living with someone with Type 1 diabetes were the same.

If you are dating, there are two things you might consider to protect yourself while out on a date. First, make sure you have some kind of diabetes identification—either a medical identification bracelet or a card in your wallet. Second, you might think about being pickier about where you go to eat on the first few dates. For example, if pizza usually causes your blood sugar to spike, it would be best to avoid it on a date, so you can feel your best and not have to deal with a high blood sugar mid-date.

One important conversation that you will need to have with your significant other is the element of accountability. Aaron cares for me deeply, and similar to my parents, wants my diabetes to be in good control. But, this concern can sometimes turn him into feeling more like a parent than a spouse. You will want to discuss this with your significant other and determine what, if any, accountability you want. (This can also be an issue with close friends, but mostly occurs with significant others due to the closer relationship.)

Because Type 1 diabetes is so exhausting and relentless, having a really good support system is important. I, unfortunately, know many people who have partners who guilt-trip them about all the costs and can't be bothered to help in any way. I'm totally self-sufficient, but I also know from experience that Aaron won't hesitate to get me a regular soda if I go low while we're out and about, for example.

Education is key when it comes to your support system, especially for those who live with you. The more equipped someone is, the more prepared they are, and they safer you will be. If someone has no interest in being educated about your diabetes or helping you, you might need to reconsider if they should be in your support system.

Parenting

Whether you have children or want children, there's something you need to know: Your diabetes won't care if it's lunchtime and the three toddlers in your kitchen are crying. Figuring out how to juggle your diabetes along with all of your normal parent activities is something that may take time.

For example, Kate Secondo is a mom of two kids who was diagnosed after her first child was born. When her children were toddlers they really didn't understand why Kate got to eat candy or drink a juice box, and would cry because they wanted some. So, she decided to only treat her lows with Hot Tamales candy. The first time she used them during a low blood sugar, Kate got the usual whining, so she gave her kids each one Hot Tamale. Of course, they thought they were terrible, and that put an end to that problem! Now that her kids are 7 and 11, Kate still only uses Hot Tamales. It's an unspoken rule that if the kids find Hot Tamales around the house, in the car, or in a purse, they are only for Kate.

Making your kids aware of your diabetes is also something you'll need to consider. Mary Ellen Phipps is also a mom of two, and her Type 1 diabetes has always been a part of the dialogue with her daughters. They know Mary Ellen has diabetes and that she has to wear a "medicine patch." But, Mary Ellen tries to be careful about how she talks about her diabetes in front of her daughters, and really only says she feels "sick" around them when her blood sugar is low.

As her daughters have gotten older, they've learned that when Mary Ellen says she feels sick, that it means Mommy needs a minute to rest and eat a snack.

Telling your children about your diabetes might start with something as simple as saying, "I have something called Type 1 diabetes, and I have to take medicine when I eat." As they get older and can understand more, you could further explain insulin, blood sugars, and so forth. Especially if you are a single parent, you want your children to know the signs of low and high blood sugars, how to check your blood sugar, how to treat a low blood sugar, how to call 911, and what to tell a 911 dispatcher.

There are some precautions you can take to protect yourself, especially if you have periods of time when you're home alone with your kids:

- Get a CGM, and have your partner or a family member "follow" your CGM through the app. This allows your partner or family member to see your blood sugars at all times.
- Talk to your kids about your diabetes, and train them to call 911 and what to say if you have passed out.
- When they're old enough, teach your kids how to administer a glucagon shot.

Bailey Ketterl's two daughters each know how to call 911 or to go get the neighbors if something happens to her. Bailey's husband is in the military, so he is sometimes gone for extended periods of time. During those times, Bailey makes it a point to check in with her family more frequently.

Every situation is different, so it's important that you have a safety plan in place to protect yourself.

Action Steps

1. If you live alone, decide what safety precautions you will put in place.
2. If you're dating someone or married, take some time to talk about your diagnosis, and how they can best help you moving forward.
3. If you're a parent, come up with a game plan for how and when you will tell your kids about your diagnosis.

Chapter 5
Health and Fitness

...

Weight Loss

Whether they're dealing with Type 1 diabetes or not, millions of people want to lose weight for one reason or another. Trying to lose weight as someone with Type 1 diabetes may be difficult. This, in part, is because insulin prevents the breakdown of fat cells and stimulates the creation of body fat. This does not mean that insulin is literally making you fatter when you take your insulin; insulin just makes weight loss a little complicated. In fact, if you have just been diagnosed in the last few weeks, there's a chance you may notice some weight gain over the next few months.

If you research how people with Type 1 diabetes can try to lose weight, you'll probably come across a low-carb, high-fat diet (LCHF). Similarly, there is also a ketogenic diet, which has stricter guidelines than just eating foods that are low-carb. The reason so many people with Type 1 diabetes are drawn to these diets is that if you eat fewer carbs throughout the day, you won't need to take as much insulin. Individuals with Type 1 diabetes take insulin based on how many carbs they eat, but there are foods that are extremely low-carbohydrate—meats and vegetables, mainly. That being said, there are some people with Type 1 diabetes may also require insulin when eating protein or fat. Your doctor can discuss this with you.

Both of these diets should be approached with extreme caution. Please remember it's important to consult your physician before changing your diet or eating habits, especially if you have any other medical conditions or are pregnant.

Following a low-carb diet is not the only option for losing weight. Working with a personal trainer and/or registered dietitian to help you lose weight could be something to consider. I have worked with a personal trainer for a few years to help me get in better shape and lose weight. I was not put on any type of restrictive diet and have still been able to lose weight.

If you are looking to modify any recipes, consider using substitutes like almond or coconut flour. There are also many baking recipes that use ingredients like avocados or sugar-free applesauce. Though you may not actually need to follow a specific meal plan, looking into ketogenic, vegan, or paleo recipes could be helpful in maintaining better blood sugar control. Like I mentioned previously, it's all about knowing which foods wreak havoc on your blood sugars.

Diabetes and Working Out

Being physically active can help with weight loss, and improved overall health, but exercise can also cause low blood sugars. This can make playing sports or working out when you have Type 1 diabetes a little challenging—not impossible, just challenging. I always played volleyball growing up and now work out at the gym several days a week.

Before you begin playing any sports or working out, it's important to talk to your doctor. Get an idea of how long workouts will last and what they might entail. With this information in hand, you can form a game plan for how to adjust snacks and insulin levels before and after your physical activity.

It is a tricky situation when you mix food, exercise, and insulin. Exercise lowers blood sugars, but food raises blood sugars. There may be a lot of trial and error, so open communication with your doctor will be important.

Asher Okin was an avid runner before being diagnosed as an individual with Type 1 diabetes, running a handful of half-marathons and a full marathon, along with 5K and 10K races. Getting back into running after his diagnosis was difficult, especially while on insulin shots, because he didn't adjust his long-acting basal at first. Eventually, Asher switched to using an insulin pump and CGM, and now schedules his workouts in the morning to leverage his increased morning insulin resistance.

Allison Caggia has Type 1 diabetes and competes in amateur CrossFit competitions just for fun. To keep her blood sugars in check, she eats a low-carb meal before a competition. Allison realized that high-intensity interval workouts and weightlifting would cause her blood sugars to spike after the workout, so she now takes one unit of insulin just minutes before she begins a workout, so that the insulin starts to kick in toward the end of her workout and bring her blood sugar back into the normal range.

Again, it may feel like you have to put everything on hold after your diagnosis. Not true! Many professional athletes are active with Type 1 diabetes: Jay Cutler was an NFL quarterback, Gary Hall, Jr. was an Olympic gold-medal swimmer, and Kelli Kuehne was an American pro golfer. It's safe to say that professional athletes endure more physical activity than the rest of us.

It takes everyone some trial and error to figure out what works before, during, and after exercise. The most important thing is to always have insulin on hand in case of high blood sugars, and glucose tabs or some kind of sugar on hand to treat low blood sugars. If you are nervous about your blood sugars and exercise, start with something low-key like riding a bike around your neighborhood.

Pregnancy

As of the writing of this book, I have not had children, but my mom did talk to me about pregnancy when I was younger. While I was definitely not planning on having children at that age, she talked to me—warned me—about the importance of good blood sugar control before and during pregnancy.

If possible, before you become pregnant, talk with your endocrinologist. This is important so that your endocrinologist can evaluate the current state of your diabetes and give you the "okay" to conceive. You will also want to find an OB-GYN who has experience with pregnancies and mothers who have Type 1 diabetes.

Jessica Betzing, who has had diabetes for more than 20 years and has one daughter, said that it's important to remember that you know your body and how your body behaves with diabetes. You have a voice—a very important voice—and shouldn't ever let anyone override your own instinct.

Contrary to what you might have read online or seen in movies like *Steel Magnolias,* many women can safely have children of their own. It's more than possible, but it does take work and extra care. Morning sickness or a general inability to keep food down causes low blood sugars, and intense cravings for weird food can cause high blood sugars, but what's most important is that your blood sugars don't stay there. One of the most important details is to consistently maintain a healthy blood sugar level. According to the American Diabetes Association, women with poorly controlled blood sugars put themselves and their babies at risk for more complications.

Kate Secondo, whom you read about in Chapter 4, developed Type 1 diabetes after her first pregnancy. She shared that diabetic pregnancy was really difficult. The first trimester brought many scary lows. After the first trimester, she followed a paleo diet. During the third trimester, she was so insulin-resistant that she was taking more than 100 units of insulin a day on a low-carb diet (compared to her usual 20–25 units of insulin a day on a moderate-carb diet).

Kate's insurance company would not cover a CGM during her pregnancy, so she tested her blood sugar every hour while awake and set an alarm to test every two hours while she slept. She did this to keep her A1C in the high 5s throughout her pregnancy. A healthy A1C during pregnancy helps keep the baby healthy as well.

During her pregnancy, Kate saw her regular OB-GYN, a high-risk OB-GYN, her endocrinologist, and her primary care doctor. All of her doctors wanted to see Kate frequently throughout her pregnancy, so much so that she had four doctors' appointments a week toward the end of her pregnancy.

Heather Wilkins also saw both a maternal-fetal medicine specialist and her OB-GYN throughout her pregnancy. A maternal-fetal medicine specialist is a doctor who specializes in high-risk pregnancies, like women who have Type 1 diabetes. Heather struggled with a lot of low blood sugars in her first trimester, but then struggled with insulin resistance. She was taking 200–230 units of insulin per day during her last trimester. With the help of Heather's insulin pump and CGM, and taking Metformin, she was able to maintain an A1C of 5.2 throughout her pregnancy.

It's not just pregnancy, but also postpartum that can affect your diabetes. Heather dealt with frequent low blood sugars, going from 200–230 units per day to 60–80 units per day—literally overnight. Another factor that affected Heather's blood sugars was breastfeeding, so eventually she decided, for her own physical health and mental health, that they needed to switch to formula. As a mom, never forget that your own health is just as important as the baby's health.

Bailey Ketterl, whom you also read about in Chapter 4, had an experience similar to Heather's, in which she had to cut her basal rates in half after she gave birth. Bailey shared that while breastfeeding both of her daughters, she had to give very little insulin for food, because her body was adjusting to all of the changes. It took her about three weeks to fine-tune her basal and bolus rates, so give yourself and your body plenty of time to adjust!

There are two things that all of these women have in common: They have Type 1 diabetes, and they have healthy, thriving children. While handling pregnancy and your Type 1 diabetes might require some extra attention and care, it's totally doable. As I mentioned previously, you'll want to work closely with your team of doctors to get the best care for you and your baby.

Mental Health: Depression and Burnout

Having diabetes has always affected my self-image, but the hardest part of living with Type 1 diabetes is that it has affected, and will always affect, my family and our day-to-day lifestyle. Type 1 diabetes is a team effort, and there's guilt that comes with it, knowing I'm adding extra stress to others' lives. Not to mention, those with diabetes are always thinking about what could go wrong next week, next year, or in 10 years—without trying to totally lose hope. It's a stress that only other individuals with Type 1 diabetes understand.

Doctors don't always tell you about the mental and emotional toll that this disease can take on you and your family. Diabetes burnout is a very real thing. You may not experience it for several years, but it's something you need to be aware of. William Polonsky's book *Diabetes Burnout: What to Do When You Can't Take it Anymore* is a great in-depth resource on this subject.

Keeping Type 1 diabetes in consistent, good control takes a lot of intentional effort—and it can be exhausting. After many, many years, sometimes people with Type 1 diabetes lose the motivation to keep everything in good control.

During a period of burnout, people with Type 1 diabetes can begin to ignore certain parts of their care (checking blood sugars less often, not taking insulin, etc.).

Burnout is important to address, because it could potentially also lead to depression. According to the American Diabetes Association, there is no definitive link between diabetes and depression, but people with Type 1 diabetes are at a higher risk for developing depression. As someone who has suffered with depression unrelated to my diabetes, I can attest to the fact that depression, regardless of the reason, can affect your diabetes management.

Experiencing burnout and depression can also lead to people with Type 1 diabetes not feeling up for the fight. While I've never personally experienced this high level of burnout, I have heard of others who have. It's difficult for them to even want to get out of bed. You may think this just sounds like depression, but it reaches another level of danger when someone with Type 1 diabetes doesn't want to get out of bed to treat a low blood sugar.

One way to help yourself during a period of burnout is to limit the number of decisions you have to make in a day. This practice also lends itself to helping you avoid something called decision fatigue. Coined by psychologist Roy F. Baumeister, decision fatigue is something many people experience after they make decision after decision all day, and eventually become so tired of making decisions that they start making poor decisions or feel they can't make a decision at all. For example, have you ever come home from work, and had no idea what you want for dinner, and can't make a decision because your brain just feels . . . empty? It's likely you're experiencing decision fatigue.

As individuals with Type 1 diabetes, we have even more decisions to make throughout each day than others do. Do I want to count this lunch as 30 carbs or 40 carbs? Should I eat cheese or crackers before my workout? Should I change my pump site before or after dinner? One way that my husband and I cut down on daily decisions is meal prepping. Every Saturday, we fix our meals for the week, and eat the same breakfast, lunch, dinner, and snacks for one week. So, I might decide that for one week, I will eat a burrito bowl for lunch every day. I'll figure out the serving sizes of each ingredient and add up the carbs so I know how much insulin to take at lunch. Then, for the rest of the week, I don't really have to put much thought to my lunch bolus, since I know it will be the same every day.

Another thing that can help prevent burnout from occurring is having "off" days built into your year. Since I was diagnosed so young, my doctors advised my parents to give me three or four days a year to just be a kid. Halloween,

Thanksgiving, Christmas, and my birthday were our chosen "off" days, and I was allowed to eat more sweets than normal. Being older now, I have a little more flexibility in what I can eat and don't really need these "off" days.

Another pseudo-holiday that I started celebrating in college was my "diabetic birthday" (sometimes called a *dia-versary*). Growing up, each year on July 4th, my parents would say something about it being my diabetic birthday, but there was no celebration. Thanks to social media, I noticed that my friends who also had diabetes were celebrating their diabetic birthday (something like going out for dinner or getting ice cream). Now, every year I do the same. I choose to celebrate this day because it marks another year of hard work and, honestly, survival. This is a simple tradition you could start yourself!

Even with all of these strategies, you still may experience anxiety and depression. There's no shame in seeking professional help, or taking anti-anxiety or antidepressant medications. You need to take care of yourself, both physically and mentally.

Why Me?

"Why me?"

This may be a question you've already asked or one you'll ask in the future. Unfortunately, there's no great answer. It's important to remember that it's not your fault.

I still believe this, and I believe that anyone living with Type 1 diabetes will be stronger, smarter, and more independent. While I still get frustrated with diabetes from time to time, I stopped asking, "Why me?" when I came to accept my condition. Acceptance came with age, more independence in my care, and some professional counseling.

How long it takes you to accept your diagnosis will vary; there's no right or wrong time line. You might be okay with it right away. You may experience anger or grief during the first few months or years of your diagnosis. Type 1 diabetes brings a lot of changes with it, which can be overwhelming and frustrating.

With all of the changes happening, it might feel like you have to put your life on hold. You can still travel, you can still go to college football games, you can still go out with friends on a Saturday night. It just takes a little bit of extra planning.

Nat Strand won *The Amazing Race,* Crystal Bowersox almost won *American Idol,* and Nick Jonas is a successful singer and actor. It's safe to assume these individuals are independently managing their Type 1 diabetes. If they can do it, so can you.

Changing Your Mindset: It's Just a Check

Part of the everyday—more like *all day, every day*—routine for individuals with Type 1 diabetes is checking our blood sugar. At a minimum, we're supposed to check our blood sugars four times per day. Doctors typically recommend checking before each meal and before going to sleep.

Every person has their own preferences for checking blood sugars. Some only use certain fingers for the test. (I can't use my index finger or thumbs, for example.) Some use no fingers at all and use their arms for the test. Everyone tends to develop a preference for a certain glucometer brand. (There is always the chance that your insurance provider will decide it likes another glucometer brand, and your preferred brand may not be covered any longer.)

When it comes to checking my blood sugar consistently, I struggle—but not because it hurts or it's too time-consuming. I struggle because for so many years, this check was more like a pass/fail test. People use both the terms *check* and *test* when talking about this process with our glucometer. I've had to intentionally focus on changing my vocabulary to only call it a blood sugar check. Though it was never talked about in this way, my family's reactions to my blood sugar levels made it feel like a pass/fail test. A good blood sugar meant I was a good diabetic. A high or low blood sugar meant I was a bad diabetic—a bad person.

If we take this train of thought a step further, many people try not to even call someone with Type 1 diabetes a diabetic. I am not a diabetic wife, or a diabetic athlete, or a diabetic daughter. I am a wife, an athlete, a daughter— and I also happen to have Type 1 diabetes. For that reason, you'll notice that I limited the use of the word *diabetic* in this book.

You might need to have conversations with your friends and family, to remind them that you are more than your blood sugars. Even as an adult, it can be easy for parents or partners to always ask about how your blood sugars have been lately. With my own family and friends who have Type 1 diabetes, I make an effort to not have my first question always be about their blood sugars.

Action Steps

1. Make a note to track any fluctuations in your blood sugars and what may have caused the change. This can be especially helpful around the holidays or special events, so you know how certain treats affect you.

2. Start trying some different recipes for treats so that you have a few favorites to pick from to take to parties and other occasions when one might be needed.

3. In your calendar or planner, write down your date of diagnosis, so you can celebrate your "diabetic birthday" next year. If you use Google Calendar, you can make the event automatically repeat each year, so you never forget.

Chapter 6
Traveling

...

On the way home from a yearbook workshop in high school, we stopped at Sonic to get lunch. We got our food and continued home because I had a softball game to play in that evening. Little did I know, the Diet Dr Pepper I ordered turned out to not be diet after all. Drinking 32 ounces of regular Dr Pepper wreaks havoc on blood sugars. Luckily, I didn't go into DKA, as that would have meant a hospital visit. I did feel nauseous, though, and I scared my yearbook advisor half to death.

Getting the wrong drink again has happened at fast-food restaurants a few times. They confirm the drink order before handing it to my husband or me, but that still doesn't guarantee it will be right. Sometimes when a drink tastes off, I use my glucometer to "test" the drink. Instead of sticking a drop of blood on the strip, I use a drop of soda. If the glucometer reads "HI," it means my soda is not diet.

When this happens, I call the restaurant and kindly let them know what happened. To most people, a wrong drink order is just an annoyance, but it can have severe consequences for someone with Type 1 diabetes.

Simple situations like this happening close to home can make traveling with Type 1 diabetes seem scary. What else could happen when you're eating at new restaurants or visiting a foreign country?! But, it's not impossible. I've taken international vacations, gone on mission trips with lots of activity, visited amusement parks, and everything in between. Like everything else, you will be used to the travel prep after a few trips!

Keep in mind that a time change may cause a few problems with your blood sugars. Depending on how big the time change is, you might see a small spike in your blood sugars. Time changes can cause problems, for example, if your blood sugars are lower in the afternoon and your insulin pump settings are set accordingly. When your pump thinks it's the afternoon but it's actually late in the evening, it could cause a high blood sugar due to the lower insulin levels. If a trip will be longer than two days, I usually keep my insulin pump clock the same for the first day, and then adjust the time to match the time where I'm visiting. This is definitely a situation that you want to talk to your doctor about before leaving for your trip.

Air Travel

As someone who flies a few times a year, I'll warn you that most airport security agents believe an insulin pump and continuous glucose monitor (CGM) can go through a body scanner, while most insulin pump manufacturing companies say they can't.

Specifically, here are the airport guidelines for a few different devices:

- Medtronic's website states, "You can continue to wear your insulin pump or continuous glucose monitor (CGM) while going through common security systems such as an airport metal detector as it will not harm the device or trigger an alarm. Do not send the devices through the x-ray machine. You need to remove your insulin pump and CGM (sensor and transmitter) while going through an airport body scanner."

- Omnipod's website states, "Pod and PDMs can safely pass through airport X-ray machines. The Pod and PDM can tolerate common electromagnetic and electrostatic fields, including airport security and cellular phones."

- Tandem's website states, "Tandem insulin pump should NOT be put through machines that use

X-rays, including airline luggage X-ray machines and full-body scanners."

- Dexcom's website states, "When wearing your G6, ask for hand-wanding or a full-body pat down and visual inspection instead of going through the Advanced Imaging Technology (AIT) body scanners (also called a millimeter wave scanner). Don't put your Dexcom G6 CGM System components through x-ray machines."

- Freestyle Libre's website states, "Some airport full-body scanners include x-ray or millimeter radio-wave, which you cannot expose your System to. The effect of these scanners has not been evaluated and the exposure may damage the System or cause inaccurate results."

So, it's safe to say that it's recommended to only go through a metal detector with your pump or CGM, or get a pat-down from the TSA. I find it easiest to always allow for a little extra time and request a pat-down during each visit to the airport.

If you do not have a pump or CGM, TSA regulations state that you will need to carry your syringes and insulin vials *together* with a pharmacy label that clearly identifies the medication. Never store insulin in checked luggage, because it may be exposed to extreme (often freezing) temperatures, which can change its effectiveness. It's also better to have it in your carry-on so, if the airline loses your luggage, you still have your insulin. You'll also want to carry your glucagon in its pharmacy-labeled container. If you are bringing extra lancets, they will need to be capped and carried along with your glucometer. Should you have any difficulties when trying to pass through airport security, Medtronic's website recommends you ask to speak with the TSA ground security commissioner.

I've traveled internationally without problems, but not everyone is as lucky. Heather Wilkins, whom you might remember from Chapter 4, had to take a trip to the emergency room while visiting London, because she got the flu. Luckily, she was able to receive some medicine to help her recover for her trip back to the States. During that visit she learned that people with Type 1 diabetes in America use different units when measuring blood sugar levels than those living in Europe. According to the American Diabetes Association, most blood sugar test results are reported as mmol/L (millimoles per liter) outside of the United States. In the United States, blood sugars are shown as mg/dL (milligrams per deciliter).

Ellie Hook, my camp friend whom I mentioned previously, has traveled abroad several times and also hasn't always had the best luck. In fact, once her insulin pump stopped working right before she ventured into the Amazon rainforest. Because there are so many barriers to getting a new pump while abroad (phoning an international number, time differences, short stays at one address, language barriers, etc.), she tried to get long-acting insulin at a local pharmacy to supplement her short-acting insulin and used manual shots for the duration of the trip. Simultaneously, she had the manufacturing company ship a replacement pump to her home address so it would be waiting for her when she returned. (Most insulin pump companies will actually provide a backup pump for international travel to take with you. You just call to make the arrangements ahead of time.)

Packing for Your Trip

When I was younger, I took three bags on every trip: my suitcase, my glucometer and insulin purse, and a soft cooler bag for snacks. There are several things to consider while you're packing and planning.

Snacks

You will need some snacks to have on hand during your trip. You'll want a variety of snacks, but don't forget to have some kind of protein snack. Cheese sticks and beef jerky are great options because they aren't messy. Peanut butter is a good option to have available for when you are back at the hotel.

Cooler

Insulin, glucometers, and test strips need to stay at room temperature. If you're also storing drinks and have ice packs in the cooler, do not allow any of the medical supplies to touch the ice packs. You could potentially keep your medical supplies in the cooler, as long as they don't directly touch the ice. If you get out of the car at a rest stop or restaurant, be sure to take all the medical supplies inside with you so that they don't get too hot or cold.

Sugar

Inevitably, your blood sugar will go low, so you need to have some kind of sugar on hand. Juice boxes are great for the car or a hotel room. If you'll be out and about, juice boxes aren't as handy, so try to have glucose tablets or hard candy. Depending on where you'll be, you might be able to run into a convenience store or restaurant and grab a regular soda, too. I always buy a bottle of regular soda before I get on an airplane, so that I have something for the flight, as well as during the car ride from the airport to the hotel.

Diabetes Supplies

You will, of course, need a glucometer, pump supplies, CGM supplies, test strips, insulin bottles (or pens), and needles. If you are on an insulin pump, also want to take extra insulin needles, in case the pump stops working during your trip. You also want to be sure and include your glucagon.

Always be sure to take *extra* pump supplies, because you never know when bad weather might strike and keep you from getting home on time. Most home pharmacies can (and will) send a prescription to wherever you are, but that won't help when it comes to insulin pump supplies. If you are going overseas and you wear an insulin pump, I recommend also getting a long-acting insulin (like Lantus) to also have on hand.

Doctor's Note

If you are traveling overseas, carry a doctor's note that says you have Type 1 diabetes and need the medical supplies that you are carrying with you. Airport security agents may not even ask for it or look for it, but better safe than sorry. A letter isn't necessary when traveling domestically but is still recommended as a precaution.

Diabetes and Driving

It's always a smart idea to check your blood sugar before getting behind the wheel. It's never safe for you to drive while your blood sugar is out of range, especially if it is low. This is especially true because if you are low and pulled over by a police officer, there is a chance they could be accused of driving under the influence, since the symptoms of low blood sugar and being intoxicated are very similar.

You should always keep something in the car to treat low blood sugars (glucose tabs, Gatorade, granola bars, peanuts, etc.). My purse is always full of hard candies, the middle console in my car contains snacks, and I have additional snacks in my trunk. I also keep spare change in my car in case I run out of treatment options in my car and need to buy something. (I do have a debit card, but I keep change on hand in case my only option is a vending machine.)

Every state has different licensing laws and policies for people with Type 1 diabetes. You can easily look up this information on the American Diabetes Association website.

Action Steps

1. Buy a bag (or two) to carry your supplies with you when needed. Check www.thetype1life.com for resources.
2. If you have a pump or CGM, check the manufacturer's website to review their airport security recommendations.
3. Create a go-to checklist on your phone or on your computer to reference each time you pack for a trip.

Chapter 7
Diabetes in the Workplace

...

My own experience, and talking with many other people who have diabetes, shows it is more than possible to have a full-time job with minimal disruptions from diabetes. After college, I worked at four different organizations and never had a major issue at work. Ironically, I now work for myself, and there have been a handful of times when I've had a low blood sugar happen during a client phone call—luckily nothing too serious, but still a bit problematic. (I've also had a few low blood sugars while writing this book!)

I recommend having a bin or drawer at work for supplies (extra test strips, extra pump supplies, glucose tabs, hard candies, packets of honey, granola bars, etc.). As I mentioned previously, you always want to be prepared. You never know when the vending machine at work will break down, and you don't want to be left stranded without treatment options. I even recommend bringing a small juice or some hard candies into long meetings, so you can treat a low blood sugar without having to leave.

Protecting Yourself at Work with the Americans with Disabilities Act (ADA)

While most employers are considerate of the needs of those who have diabetes at work, there's always the chance that you may have difficulties with the way your employer responds to your diabetes. This could mean problems with how often you have low blood sugars, problems with the noise of your devices, or even problems with having a diabetic alert dog.

Accommodations

If you have a job with physical activity or limited breaks during work hours, your employer is required to provide reasonable accommodations, something you can talk to your HR department or representative about. According to the ADA, examples of reasonable accommodations may include privacy to check your blood sugar, breaks for snacks, or slight changes to shift times. Your employer is not required to oblige to every accommodation request, especially if it's one that is difficult to accommodate or expensive.

Privacy

A potential employer cannot ask you if you have diabetes during an interview, nor are you required to disclose it. But after making a job offer, an employer may ask questions about your health and can even require a medical exam, as long as all applicants for the same type of job are asked the same questions and required to get an exam.

You may think that it's not necessary to tell your coworkers or your boss because you are an adult and have things under control. Informing some of your colleagues about your diabetes is a smart idea to protect yourself, though. Sudden spikes or blood sugar drops can happen to anyone, at any time. If your blood sugar drops while you're at work, you could pass out or make an error in your work.

You could start with one person and slowly tell others as you become more comfortable. This will also depend on the size of your company or department. If you're one of 100, it may make sense to only tell your closest friends at work. But, if you work on a small team of seven every day, it might make the most sense to tell everyone. If you haven't already experienced this, you'll soon realize that almost everyone knows someone who has diabetes, so most people are already familiar with it.

What's important to remember is that you are in control of who you tell and when. It's not legal for your boss to disclose your diagnosis to your coworkers without your consent. According to the ADA, your boss is only allowed to disclose your diagnosis to supervisors who need medical information in order to provide you any necessary accommodations.

Ellie Hook, whom I've mentioned in previous chapters, shared that she's always approached telling her coworkers about her diabetes as it comes up naturally. Often, people in the office will notice her checking her blood sugar or taking insulin, which starts the conversation.

Medical Leave

As you know, you can't drive while your blood sugar is low. So, going low right as you need to leave for work can be quite problematic. Even worse, you may end up in the hospital with DKA and need to miss a few days of work.

Depending on your employer, you could be protected by the Family and Medical Leave Act (FMLA). According to the U.S. Department of Labor, FMLA allows eligible employees to take up to 12 workweeks of unpaid, job-protected leave for certain family and medical reasons, including serious health problems that makes the employee unable to perform the essential functions of his or her job.

But, if your employer has a reasonable belief that you may be unable to perform your job, the employer may ask for a note from your doctor. For example, if you need to adjust your hours because of the current state of your diabetes, your employer may ask you to provide a doctor's note indicating there are limits on how many hours a day you can work.

Alert Dogs

Lauren Burke, whom you met in Chapter 2 and who has a diabetic alert dog, was very open at work from the beginning about her Type 1 diabetes and her dog. She even gave a presentation to everyone on her first day at a new job, explaining diabetes, her alert dog, Ricki, and how people should behave around Ricki. Lauren shared that her coworkers really struggled with the "no touch, no talk, no eye contact" rule, but eventually they got it.

When Lauren moved to another job, she ran into some problems. The building management company told Lauren she couldn't have Ricki in most parts of the building—which is illegal. To make matters worse, they also said she could only relieve Ricki in a particular spot outside. It's important to know your rights, and the ADA allows an alert dog to accompany its owner into all public places, including restaurants, stores, and schools.

Discrimination at Work

Unfortunately, you may encounter discriminatory circumstances at your job. This could look like your boss not giving you extra shifts, being forced to take your shots in the bathroom, or being wrongly fired while in the hospital. There are a few resources that can help you.

Job Accommodation Network (JAN)
JAN offers free, expert, and confidential guidance on workplace accommodations and disability employment issues. JAN helps both people with disabilities (including Type 1 diabetes) and employers with employees that have disabilities. JAN has information about accommodation ideas for people with Type 1.

WorkplaceFairness.org
Workplace Fairness is a nonprofit that helps promote and preserve employees rights. They have information on everything from discrimination, benefits, unions, harassment, and when/how to pursue legal action.

U.S. Equal Employment Opportunity Commission (EEOC)
The EEOC is responsible for enforcing federal laws that make it illegal to discriminate against a job applicant or an employee for a few different reasons, including disability.

Their website includes a lot of information regarding the Americans with Disabilities Act (ADA).

If you experience discrimination, there are actions you can take. For example, if your boss or a colleague makes rude comments about treating a low blood sugar at your desk, talk to someone in human resources or, if you are part of a union, your union rep. Depending on the size of your company, HR could have your boss or colleagues take a diabetes educational course.

Protecting Yourself while Working from Home

If you work remotely for a company, or run your own business from home, you may not have to worry about telling coworkers or having a meeting with HR. In Chapter 4, I talked about how to protect yourself if you live alone. Similarly, if you work remotely, think about what kind of safety precautions you can take to protect yourself. Even though I'm married, I spend most of my days alone and sometimes worry about my blood sugar dropping too low. Here are a few things you could do:

- Introduce yourself to your neighbors, and give one of them a spare key into your house or apartment. Obviously, this would really only be helpful if your neighbors also work from home, don't work, or are retired.

- Get a CGM, and have friends and family in the area "follow" your CGM through the app.
- If you don't have a team, find some virtual work friends! Running my own business, I don't work on a team, but I do have business friends that I talk with regularly—so much so that they might sense something is wrong if they don't hear from me every few hours.
- Wear a Life Alert® necklace around the house.
- Make sure to have low blood sugar treatment supplies in various rooms/places around your house or apartment, so you're never too far away from them. I always have snacks or juice at my desk, especially when I'm going to be on calls with clients.
- Instead of working from home alone, rent an office at a coworking space nearby. Or, opt to spend your days working from a coffee shop or the library.

Action Steps

1. Set up a meeting with your boss or HR department to discuss your diagnosis and what accommodations you might need.
2. Keep some low blood sugar treatment options in your workspace.

Conclusion

...

So, now what? What do you do next?

Focus on what can, or does, go right. So much of our time as individuals with Type 1 diabetes is already spent thinking about what can go wrong or listening to our doctors lecture us about what we're doing wrong.

While I do still struggle with guilt sometimes, as I mentioned previously, I understand as an adult that, while it was sometimes a challenge for others, it wasn't a burden because they love me. My hope in sharing some of these experiences is that you can realize the same thing.

Take it a day at a time. That may sound cliche, but it's some of the best advice when dealing with diabetes. As mentioned, there are patterns you may notice in your blood sugars, but doing the same thing day after day can still yield different results. You may have weeks when your sugars are all over the place, which can be overwhelming and frustrating. So, focus on today.

You feel overwhelmed right now and might be wondering, *How will I figure out the next 10 or 20 years?* It will get easier. It may not ever be *easy*, but it will get *easier*. Don't give in. You might feel like you are losing the battle, like you are overwhelmed, like you just can't keep it up. I mentioned that you might need to see a counselor at some point, and I strongly consider trying it. Work through your emotions, instead of suppressing your feelings.

If you have a problem or a question, call someone and get the answer. Never feel like you are a bother to anyone; this is your life. So if you need help, call as many doctors, nurses, help lines, or other adults with the same issues as you need to until you get a satisfactory answer. When I was a kid, my dad sometimes joked that the staff at the doctor's office was probably looking at the caller ID and playing rock, paper, scissors to see who got to answer his and my mom's next question.

Lastly, know that you will make it through this and be better for it. I hate math, but I can calculate the carbs in almost any food at the drop of a hat, in my head. I'm resilient and adapt to change fairly easily. Who knew that a 3-year-old, diagnosed with Type 1 diabetes 26 years ago, would be writing this book for you to read to help you navigate life with your own diabetes?

What might you be doing 20 years from now to impact others?

Resources

For these resources and more, visit www.thetype1life.com.

American Diabetes Association
www.diabetes.org

JDRF
www.jdrf.org

Beyond Type 1
www.beyondtype1.org

Diabetes Daily
www.diabetesdaily.com

T1 Everyday Magic
www.t1everydaymagic.com

Diabetes Burnout: What to Do When You Can't Take it Anymore
by William Polonsky

Dr. Bernstein's Diabetes Solution: A Complete Guide to Achieving Normal Blood Sugars
By Richard K. Bernstein, www.diabetes-book.com

MySugr: Diabetes Tracker Log
www.mysugr.com

MyFitnessPal
www.myfitnesspal.com

CalorieKing
www.calorieking.com

Sugarmate
www.sugarmate.io

Diabits
www.diabits.com

Job Accommodation Network (JAN)
www.askjan.org

Workplace Fairness
www.workplacefairness.org

U.S. Equal Employment Opportunity Commission (EEOC)
www.eeoc.gov

Glossary

A1C: According to the American Diabetes Association, a test that gives you a picture of your average blood glucose (blood sugar) control for the past two to three months.

Carbohydrates: According to Merriam-Webster.com, a substance (as a starch or sugar) that is rich in energy and is made up of carbon, hydrogen, and oxygen. *(These are what you take insulin for.)*

Continuous Glucose Monitor (CGM): According to Dexcom.com, an FDA-approved device that provides continuous insight into glucose levels throughout the day and night. The device displays information about glucose direction and speed providing users additional information to help with diabetes management.

Diabetic Ketoacidosis (DKA): According to Mayo Clinic, a serious complication of diabetes that occurs when your body produces high levels of blood acids called ketones.

Diabulimia: According to the National Eating Disorders Association, the reduction of insulin intake by Type 1 diabetics in an effort to lose weight.

Endocrinology: According to Merriam-Webster.com, a branch of medicine concerned with the structure, function, and disorders of the endocrine glands. *(You will visit your endocrinologist every few months to make adjustments to your diabetes care.)*

Glucagon: According to Merriam-Webster.com, a protein hormone that is produced especially by the islets of Langerhans and that promotes an increase in the sugar content of the blood by increasing the rate of glycogen breakdown in the liver. *(A glucagon kit should be kept on hand in case of severe hypoglycemia.)*

Glucometer: According to the FDA, a test system for use at home to measure the amount of sugar (glucose) in your blood. *(Also referred to as just a "meter," a glucometer should be kept near you at all times, so you can check your blood sugar at a moment's notice.)*

Glucose tabs: According to WebMD.com, chewable sugar tablets used by people with diabetes to raise their blood sugar quickly when it drops dangerously low, a condition known as hypoglycemia.

Hyperglycemia: According to Merriam-Webster.com, an excess of sugar in the blood. *(Hyperglycemia is also referred to as a "high blood sugar.")*

Hypoglycemia: According to Merriam-Webster.com, an abnormal decrease of sugar in the blood. *(Hypoglycemia is also referred to as a "low blood sugar.")*

Ketones: According to the American Diabetes Association, a chemical produced when there is a shortage of insulin in the blood and the body breaks down body fat for energy.

About the Author

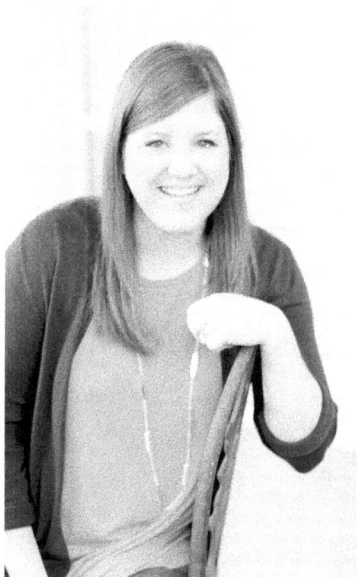

Jessica Freeman is a Type 1 diabetes advocate and has been living with Type 1 diabetes for 26 years. Jessica is also the owner of Jess Creatives, an award-winning graphic and web design company. Jessica lives in Atlanta, Georgia, with her husband, Aaron, and their cocker spaniel, Morgan Freeman.

Also from Jessica Freeman

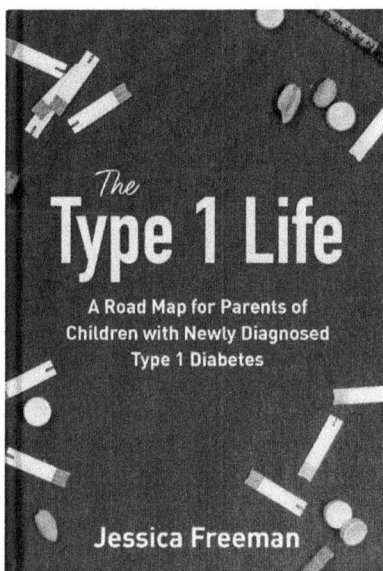

A diagnosis of Type 1 diabetes can happen at any age. If you know a child who has also been recently diagnosed with Type 1 diabetes, their family is likely feeling just as overwhelmed with what to do next. While there's nothing cookie-cutter about Type 1 diabetes management, The Type 1 Life helps parents understand how to tell friends and family about their child's diagnosis, navigate school and sports with diabetes, foster independence and self-management, and prepare their child for college and adulthood. Visit www.thetype1life.com for more info.

www.ingramcontent.com/pod-product-compliance
Lightning Source LLC
Chambersburg PA
CBHW060510280326
41933CB00014B/2912